KT-439-192

The New
Self Help Series
DANDRUFF

WITHDRAWN

The New Self Help Series

DANDRUFF
and Other Scalp Problems

LEON CHAITOW
N.D., D.O.

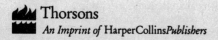

Thorsons
An Imprint of HarperCollins*Publishers*

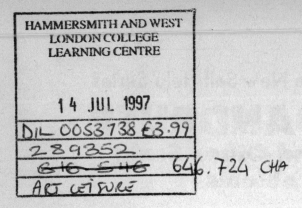

Thorsons
An Imprint of HarperCollins*Publishers*
77–85 Fulham Palace Road,
Hammersmith, London W6 8JB
1160 Battery Street,
San Francisco, California 94111–1213

Published by Thorsons 1994
1 3 5 7 9 10 8 6 4 2

A catalogue record for this book is available from the
British Library

ISBN 07225 3016 1

Printed in Great Britain by
HarperCollinsManufacturing, Glasgow

289352

Contents

Note to reader

Before following the self-help advice given in
this book, readers are earnestly urged to give careful
consideration to the nature of their particular health
problem, and to consult a competent physician if in any
doubt. This book should not be regarded as a substitute
for professional medical treatment, and whilst every
care is taken to ensure the accuracy of the content,
the author and publishers cannot accept legal
responsibility for any problem arising out of the
experimentation with the methods described.

CHAPTER ONE

What is Dandruff?

Dandruff is a scalp condition in which flakes of dead skin are shed, sometimes in great profusion. There might also be mild inflammation of the scalp leading to itching and irritation. Some experts believe that dandruff is associated with hair loss, while others believe there is no such link.

A SYMPTOM, NOT A DISEASE

While dandruff is unsightly and undoubtedly causes a great deal of embarrassment and distress, it is not a disease but merely a symptom. When there is dandruff there is also a cause – some underlying imbalance which can and should be corrected.

Most experts, such as Dr Thomas Goodman, believe that dandruff is no more than an extension to the scalp of an extremely common (usually facial) skin problem, *seborrhoeic dermatitis*. Other researchers and skin experts, such as leading British dermatologist

Dr Sam Shuster, believe that there is no doubt that dandruff is a *yeast* problem, an infection of the skin caused by fungal organisms.

The truth is that dandruff can be either a part of a more general dermatitis *or* evidence of yeast colonization, and sometimes both. The fungus now thought by medical researchers to be responsible for many cases of dandruff is *Pityrsporum*. The following chapters will help you to identify which is the case in your particular condition.

NOT JUST A LOCAL PROBLEM

In order to control and rid yourself of dandruff you need to deal with it on two levels. First, on a local level (scalp hygiene, shampoos and lotions etc.). The second level involves eliminating the reasons that allowed the dandruff to happen in the first place – systemically. By 'systemically' I mean that the underlying health of the body is what decides whether such symptoms appear, whether problems occur at all, and whether they become chronic – and it is the basic underlying causes of the problem which need addressing, not just the symptom of dandruff itself.

This is not to say that we should ignore the localized scalp condition, which is clearly important from a cosmetic and self-image point of view, but that whatever we do to the scalp itself, we should also be looking for systemic causes. This might involve any of a wide range of possibilities including identifying and dealing with allergy, toxicity, deficiency or various forms of infection. Hormonal and digestive factors may also be part of the complex picture which can emerge.

Depending upon which underlying influences we can identify, treating dandruff systemically *may* call for:

- specific changes in diet
- attention to possible allergies
- introduction of methods that reduce stress levels (stress is also sometimes a feature)
- use of herbs
- taking supplements (if needed)
- use of homoeopathy
- application of hydrotherapy methods to encourage circulation and detoxification
- attention to fungal conditions in the system
- normalization of digestive imbalances if these are contributing to the condition

WHERE DO WE START?

In order to apply the correct methods which will help your particular pattern of dandruff it is necessary to identify just what is going on. The opening chapters of the book will help you to achieve this task.

Once you know what it is you are dealing with – whether this involves deficiency, toxicity, infection, allergy or anything else – appropriate, safe, self-help means for correcting the problem will be explained, and where necessary, guidance will be given as to the sort of specialized help you might need to seek. There will also be detailed description of safe, self-help, local, treatments which can be used along with a systemic approach. One without the other is unlikely to be as effective as a combination of systemic and local self-help methods.

Dandruff – whether caused by a yeast or by the various interacting factors which bring about seborrhoeic dermatitis – is unsightly and irritating (literally and figuratively). As it tends to be chronic, it therefore requires a determined effort to get rid of the causes. Successful self-help can take time – months rather than weeks.

OTHER SCALP PROBLEMS

Chapter 9 looks at other scalp problems, and explains some of the self-help approaches that can aid in controlling them. Some of these, such as *psoriasis*, are not confined to the scalp.

Hair loss – both the normal (*baldness*) and abnormal (*alopecia*) variety – also deserves our attention since it causes a great deal of distress and anxiety, especially when it occurs in individuals who invest great importance in their personal appearance.

Another unsightly and irritating condition which can cause local hair loss is *ring-worm*. This localized fungal infection is quite distinct from any other form of fungal invasion.

HAIR AND SCALP CARE

For some people the appearance of the hair makes enormous demands on time – and their budget. The hours of washing, conditioning, drying, grooming, dressing and almost obsessive attention which hair receives give us some idea of just how important an area it is for many people. Equally, the shabby, dull, lifeless and just plain unappealing nature of the hair of others indicates just how little they care about hair (and perhaps general) appearance. Perhaps a happy medium somewhere between obsession and total uninterest is called for?

If we are to have a healthy scalp and hair, some of the many practices involved in hair grooming need to be examined. Some of the methods and materials used at home, and by professional hairdressers, can and do cause great damage to the skin of the head, and to the hair itself. Chapter 8 looks at these in more detail. It also sets out the many simple but practical ways in which we can encourage a healthy hair and scalp condition, so that your crowning glory (or, for some, at least what is left of it) can be as healthy as possible.

FIRST STEPS

The next chapters will discuss the main possible causes of dandruff – seborrhoeic dermatitis and yeast infection – and will help you to identify which, if either, is likely to be involved in your own scalp condition. Other causes – stress and food allergy – are also examined. After that, the best approaches for handling the causes of the problem will be described.

CHAPTER TWO

About Seborrhoeic Dermatitis

Seborrhoeic dermatitis (SD) is probably the commonest of all skin conditions. Almost everyone has evidence of it at some time in their life. Many experts believe that it is the main cause of dandruff. SD can be mild or severe and is almost always intermittent – it comes and goes – with its worst manifestations in the winter months.

SD varies from mild to severe. When it is mild, it takes the form of a scaly, sometimes reddened and greasy (although it looks dry) rash. When more severe, it takes the appearance of yellow crusting. SD may be very itchy or have no symptoms apart from the scaling flakes of skin, which when derived from the scalp are called dandruff. If there is no obvious irritation or itching, the only signs you may notice of having dandruff could be a mantle of white flakes on the neck and shoulders of your clothes, pillows and headrests. Scratching (to be avoided if at all possible) will increase the shedding of white scaly flakes even more.

Most people with dandruff also have some degree of SD in other areas, at least for part of the year, or under particular circumstances (see below). It is therefore necessary to examine SD in a little detail so that you can identify which factors (if any) apply to you.

SD can affect the face (mainly the eyebrow area, sides of the nose and cheeks, chin and forehead) as well as behind (and in) the ears, between the shoulder blades, under the arms, in the centre of the chest and under the breasts (in women), in the groin – and, of course, on the scalp. Although commonest either in babies or at puberty, SD can begin at any age, and may not make its first appearance until middle age or later.

When it affects babies (often as soon as a few days after birth), SD is referred to as 'cradle cap'. This scaly, often brownish, dandruff-like rash is often classified as a fungal condition – and this may give a clue to the cause of adult forms of SD as well.

WHAT CAUSES SD?

The many possible causes of SD are listed below, together with conditions that are linked to SD.

Excessive Oil Production

An immediate cause of this widespread and commonly lifelong condition is an excessive degree of activity or inflammation in the areas of the body where natural skin oils – sebum – are most actively produced. This fact does not, however, explain *why* these areas are acting in this way. Many experts simply state the fact that it is an 'oily' problem, rather than telling you that it is a problem involving oily areas of the skin in which overlying skin may become apparently dry and flaky, trapping the excessive levels of oil that should emerge through the skin.

Hormonal Activity

There is a very definite link between SD and hormonal activity. This is demonstrated not only by the fact that the condition often starts around puberty, but also by its common increased activity around period time in women.

Acne

There is also a common connection between the activity of SD and acne, since both involve an increase in sebum production. Acne also has a bacterial involvement, however, with what seems to be a very definite link to stress and nutritional factors (although any nutrition link with acne is strongly denied by many medical experts).

Stress

Frequently mentioned by people with severe SD as

being an aggravating factor. The condition often seems to get worse soon after stress loads increase.

Food Allergy or Sensitivity

This seems to be another common feature – and is especially noticeable in the childhood forms of the condition. Research has shown that nearly three out of four babies with cradle cap eventually develop obvious food allergies before the age of ten (often also involving the skin in the form of eczema, or manifesting as asthma).

Milk and other dairy products seem to be a commonly noticed aggravating factor when food intolerance is linked to SD. This is not the only possibility, however, and careful detective work may be needed to identify culprit foods.

Nutritional Deficiencies

Deficiencies in certain nutrients are also commonly observed in cases of SD. The most significant of these are: selenium (which is widely used in anti-dandruff shampoos); vitamin E; B-complex vitamins (as well as individual B-vitamins, notably biotin, B_2, B_6 and B_{12}); and minerals (most commonly zinc).

Digestive Factors

There is often a direct connection between food

sensitivities, as mentioned earlier, and digestive problems which prevent adequate breakdown of foods. Such problems themselves may involve inadequate levels of digestive acids and enzymes. Alternatively, they may result from conditions existing in the lower digestive tract which allow particles into the bloodstream which should not be able to pass through the barrier provided by an intact mucous membrane in the intestines.

As will become clear, a variety of tactics may be needed to encourage more normal digestive and bowel function – including the possible use of supplements of 'friendly bacteria', digestive enzymes and colon cleansing.

Toxicity

The skin is one of the major organs of elimination of toxic residues which we acquire through food, water and drugs, and from the atmosphere. While not a cause of SD, toxicity can be a major influence on how well other aspects of body function, such as digestion and circulation, are working. These functions are important in helping the skin recover from its unbalanced behaviour, whether manifesting as dandruff or SD. Various general systemic and local detoxification methods will be outlined in later chapters.

IS THERE A YEAST CONNECTION?

As mentioned in chapter 1, Dr Sam Shuster, a leading British dermatologist, believes that there is overwhelming evidence in support of dandruff being a fungal infection. Many texts that do not make this link do, however, maintain that cradle cap is a fungal condition – and then go on to connect cradle cap with SD. Associated yeast-infection problems can often help to make this connection.

The questionnaire on page 13 will help you identify whether you have SD, and also whether yeast is likely to be a part of this. If this proves to you that yeast might well be a factor in your condition, then the information provided can help you get it under control.

WHERE TO BEGIN

The information given above and the following questionnaire can help you identify your condition. If you discover that not only do you have dandruff but also other evidence of seborrhoeic dermatitis, the next stage is to see which of the different factors discussed in chapter 3 are in need of your attention, starting with yeast. The next chapters will provide information on yeast; stress factors and tactics for reducing stress; on allergy and sensitivity; nutritional deficiency; digestive function; toxicity and detoxification methods.

As we work through the possibilities, and as you begin to deal with causes, so you will get closer to controlling the reasons why the skin on your scalp is behaving as it is.

QUESTIONNAIRE – HAVE YOU GOT SD?

1 Have you got dandruff?
2 Are there red, oily or scaly patches/areas on your face (behind ears, eyebrows, forehead, sides of nose, cheeks)?
3 Are there such areas in your armpits, in the middle of your chest, around the breast bone, below the breasts or on the groin?
4 If you answered yes to any of the previous three questions – are any of these areas also itchy or irritating?
5 If you answered yes to any of the first three questions – is the condition worse in the winter months?
6 If you answered yes to any of the first three questions – is the condition worse during or soon after periods of stress?
7 Have you ever been told by a health-care expert that you have seborrhoeic dermatitis?

If you answered yes to *any* of the first three questions and to *any one* of the other four questions, then you almost certainly do have SD. You should now complete the questionnaires relating to yeast in chapter 3 in order to see whether it is part of the problem.

If you do have SD, and if yeast is part of that problem, then the yeast connection is the first thing you should tackle – using also the guidelines for stress reduction, general nutritional excellence and detoxification as described in later chapters. The local scalp and hair treatments described in chapter 3 which are specifically aimed at yeast-related problems should also be started and used regularly.

IDENTIFYING THE CAUSES

If you believe you have seborrhoeic dermatitis, either based on a medical diagnosis or on the description given above, you should work your way through the various questionnaires in chapter 3. Then, where appropriate (based on the information you gain from the answers you give), you should follow the advice which is given at the end of each section.

The series of questionnaires given in the following chapter focuses attention on the key elements that determine, to a large extent, how well or how ill you are likely to be. Dandruff is not an illness but a symptom – and symptoms are nothing other than very definite signals and reminders that something is wrong. Such a reminder can trigger action which makes both the symptom (in this case dandruff/seborrhoeic dermatitis) improve as well as enhancing your overall energy, feeling of 'wellness' and resistance to infection.

The 'co-factors' of dandruff/SD include yeast infection; stress and how we handle it; food allergy/sensitivity issues; deficiencies; toxicities; and digestive imbalances. These are all addressed in the following chapters.

CHAPTER THREE

Yeast

Chronic yeast infection can cause a wide range of physical and emotional symptoms. It is a common cause of changes in digestive and other bodily functions, including that of the skin if it is present there. The subject deserves our special consideration.

There seems to be a rising tide of yeast-infection problems – especially in women but not uncommonly in men as well. Women are more likely to be affected because of hormonal fluctuations which encourage yeast activity, and because of the widespread use of contraceptive medication ('the Pill'), which further encourages yeast to become active. An underlying influence on both sexes is the use of antibiotics which damage the friendly bacteria which live in our intestines, and which are the main control factor which prevents yeast from spreading when we are healthy. These factors, together with a diet very high in sugar (a modern phenomenon), seem to be the key reasons for the sudden explosion of yeast-related health problems (often involving the yeast *Candida* albicans).

The most obvious aspects of yeast disease are seen in thrush erruptions in the mouth and throat, and in the vaginal area. A huge range of other – apparently unrelated – symptoms have, however, been found to derive from *Candida* activity in some people. These range from digestive upsets such as heartburn, diarrhoea and chronic bloating, to cystitis, skin eruptions, allergies, menstrual problems, constipation, anxiety, irritability and depression.

As with seborrhoeic dermatitis, systemic approaches to such conditions – as opposed to simply treating the local outbreak of infection – will get the best results. This is because when there is a local problem – say on the skin – these outbreaks are *always* associated with a widespread reservoir of yeast overgrowth in the intestinal tract – and until this is controlled the yeast will continue its activities.

DO YOU HAVE A YEAST/CANDIDA PROBLEM?

The following questionnaires will help you identify whether yeast is part of your problem.

Drug-use History

1 Have you undergone a course of antibiotic use that lasted for eight weeks or longer, or for shorter periods four or more times in one year?
2 Have you ever undergone a course of antibiotics for acne treatment for more than a month?
3 Have you been treated with steroid medication (such as cortisone or prednisone)?
4 Have you been on 'the Pill' for a year or more?
5 Have you received treatment with immuno-suppressant medication?
6 Have you been pregnant more than once?

Symptom History

1 Have you had or have you now got recurrent of persistent cystitis, vaginitis or prostatitis?
2 Have you had or have you now got endometriosis?
3 Have you had thrush (in the mouth or vagina) more than once?
4 Are you subject to athlete's foot or fungal problems with your nails or skin?
5 Do you suffer from a variety of allergies or sensitivities?
6 Are any of your symptoms worse after eating sugary or yeast-based foods, or after being exposed to chemical smells?
7 Do you suffer from abdominal bloating

regularly – or frequent diarrhoea or constipation?

8 Do you suffer from symptoms of premenstrual tension such as fluid retention?

9 Do you suffer from lethargy, exhaustion, fatigue?

10 Do you crave sweet foods or alcohol?

11 Do your muscles ache or feel tingly or numb for no obvious reason?

12 Do you suffer from impotence or lack of sexual drive?

If you answered yes to one or more of the questions in the first section, and to two or more in the second section, then you are probably suffering from yeast-related ill-health, and it could well be playing a major part in any skin or scalp problems you have.

You should apply the basic yeast treatment plan as described below *as a first priority*. Additionally, you should look carefully at the questionnaires and guidelines later in this chapter relating to stress reduction, allergies, detoxification and general nutritional excellence, and follow the advice which seems to relate to your personal needs.

CONTROLLING YEAST AND DANDRUFF

The following is a basic summary of the best way of starting to control yeast.

Leading British nutritional experts, Dr Stephen Davies and Dr Alan Stewart, suggest that the best approach to dealing with dandruff may be by means of 'a general antifungal programme, particularly if combined with the use of an anti-dandruff shampoo' (*Nutritional Medicine*, Pan Books 1989).

First, it is necessary to understand that when yeast affects any part of the body, whether as a skin condition or as *Candida* (thrush) in the vagina, mouth or throat, it is already almost certainly widely active in the intestines. This is why symptoms such as digestive distress (bloating, 'acid' stomach, diarrhoea or constipation) and genitourinary problems (recurrent cystitis, vaginitis etc.) are all too common, along with mouth and throat infection by yeast. When, however, the skin is the only affected region, the yeast infection is usually less obvious.

Any local treatment focusing only on the skin, mouth (or vagina) will have limited short-term effects. It is therefore necessary to pay particular attention to the main colonies of yeast which will almost always be flourishing in the bowel. This reason for this is that everyone has some *Candida* and other yeasts living on the body, but this is usually controlled efficiently by the immune system and by huge colonies of friendly bacteria living in our intestinal tracts (including the mouth, which is the start of the intestinal tract) and on our skin. Yeast often gets out of hand, though, when antibiotics (which damage the friendly bacteria) and other medication is used too enthusiastically or too often. This is especially so if the diet is unbalanced, containing too much sugar and not enough nutrient-rich foods.

To avoid a repetitive cycle in which yeast-related outbreaks occur whenever you are under stress or the immune system is under pressure (with another infection for example), the best approach is usually a *triple attack*. The three stages are as follows:

1 You need to attempt to kill the yeast using a variety of herbal products such as garlic, caprylic acid (coconut plant extract), aloe vera juice and sometimes the herbs hydrastis and echinacea as well (these last two herbs should not be used by pregnant women).

2 At the same time, replenishment of bowel flora should be started using proven viable colonizing strains of *L. acidophilus* (for the mouth, vagina and small intestine) and *Bifidobacteria* (for the large intestine). These are the normal controlling elements for *Candida* and other yeasts which are usually damaged when antibiotics or steroid drugs (including 'the Pill') are used medically allowing the yeast to get out of hand.

3 In addition, a diet low in sugar and high in complex carbohydrates is suggested. The diet should also contain cultured (live) dairy

products unless there is an allergy to milk or its products (see page 34). Sugar is yeast's favourite food (ask anyone who makes wine or beer), and it makes sense not to feed it while you are trying to kill it with herbs (such as garlic) and friendly bacteria.

Such methods are commonly extremely successful but may take three to six months (or more) to control the yeast overgrowth completely. Skin and other local symptoms should, however, show improvement within weeks.

People with yeast problems all too often have additional food sensitivities and allergies. These can be brought about by the detrimental activity of yeast in the intestines. Once the delicate inner lining has been damaged, it is easy for undesirable substances to be absorbed, thus triggering the allergy reactions. For this reason, extra care over diet is needed. Anything that seems to provoke symptoms should be avoided – especially if it is derived from yeasts or carries moulds on its surface.

Dietary Guidelines

- Avoid all sugars, and for the first few weeks avoid fruit as well.
- Avoid aged cheeses, dried fruits, fermented products and any food derived from or containing yeast.
- Eat at least 3 ounces (85 grams) daily of fish,

poultry or lean meat (free-range only as many factory-farmed animals and fish contain large residues of antibiotics and steroids). Vegetarians can substitute this with grains and pulses or tofu (soy 'cheese').

- Eat pulses (beans, lentils) and whole grains (especially rice), and abundantly of salad or lightly cooked vegetables.
- Use fresh virgin olive oil as a dressing on vegetables daily as it has antifungal properties.
- Daily consumption of *live* cultured milk products (low-fat if possible), such as yoghurt or kefir, is extremely helpful in *Candida* conditions – but avoid these if you are dairy sensitive. Make sure that such products contain live organisms and no sugar!

Nutritional Supplements

- Caprylic acid (coconut plant extract) capsules – 2 to 4 daily with meals (Mycopryl brand made by BioCare is suggested).
- *Acidophilus* and *Bifidobacteria* (Natren or BioCare brands) – a quarter teaspoonful in tepid water of each (or one Biocare capsule) three times daily away from meals.
- Garlic (deodorized Kyolic or PureGar brands) – 3 to 6 capsules daily with food.
- Aloe vera juice – one teaspoon in small tumbler of water several times a day.

Additional help from other herbs requires expert advice.

Expect to feel slightly unwell for the first few days of an anti-yeast diet as your body has to deal with the dead yeast cells. You may have flu-like symptoms or nausea. Be patient, and stick to the programme for at least three months.

If you have any tendency to candidiasis or other infections in the mouth, take extra care over disinfecting toothbrushes. In any case, start using a new one at least once a month to prevent reinfection as brushes are a notorious haven for micro-organisms. An ideal toothpaste to use when there is mouth candidiasis is Thursday Plantation's Tea Tree Oil paste – as the essential oil it contains has strong anti-fungal properties.

Local Treatment for Scalp and Skin

There are many anti-dandruff shampoos and hair conditioners available from pharmacies and health stores. You can select one or other of these to use while undertaking the anti-yeast programme outlined above. Products based on tea tree oil are idea for local scalp care. You can either massage the essential oil into the scalp daily or use a shampoo containing the oil. When applying shampoo, you should use 'tonic friction' – rubbing the scalp with finger tips or a bristle brush in order to stimulate the circulation. You should also utilize the general hygiene and scalp-care suggestions in chapter 8 –

the text highlights wherever these have an anti-fungal potential as well as a general one.

I have given a simple but far more thorough self-help outline for dealing with *Candida* in my book *Candida Albicans – Could Yeast be Your Problem?* (Thorsons 1991).

CHAPTER FOUR

Stress

Stress can make dandruff worse – for although we tend to think of stress as affecting our emotions and 'nerves', science has shown that there is a direct link between our minds, our emotions and our defence/immune systems. People with acne, for example, have been able to rid themselves of the worst of their condition by learning deep relaxation methods; and doctors monitoring people with a tendency to recurrent herpes infections have been able to predict accurately when outbreaks will occur based only on the reported stress levels of these individuals.

If stress can influence acne and herpes infections it can certainly influence yeast infections (or rather the way our bodily controls over the yeast are operating). It can also have an effect on many of the other possible interacting causes of seborrhoeic dermatitis.

QUESTIONNAIRE

1 Do you work more than a five-and-a-half day week?

2 Do you often work more than 10 hours daily?

3 Do you rush your meal-breaks – allowing less than 30 minutes?

4 Do you eat quickly, chewing very little?

5 Are you a smoker?

6 Do you sleep less than seven hours each night?

7 Do you spend time relaxing listening to music regularly ?

8 Do you do daily relaxation exercises?

9 Do you exercise – walking or anything else – for at least 20 minutes every other day?

10 Do you have a hobby which is relaxing to you – ideally something creative (gardening, painting, knitting)?

11 Are you involved in any sporting activity which is not competitive (cycling, swimming, walking)?

12 Do you go to a yoga or exercise class regularly?

13 Do you try to take a short break, perhaps sleep, during the day?

14 Do you have some form of regular 'maintenance' treatment – massage, aromatherapy or osteopathy for example?

15 Do you get out of doors into daylight for at least half an hour a day?

The answers to questions 1 to 6 should *all* be 'no', and if you answered yes to any of them, you know what to do. The answers to questions 7 to 15 should *all* be 'yes' – and if there are some 'no' answers, try to make at least some of them 'yes' as soon as you can!

WHAT CAN YOU DO ABOUT STRESS?

- Start to alter the answers to the questions above to more appropriate ones.
- Give yourself time to learn real relaxation from books, tapes or instruction in classes (my book *The Stress-Protection Plan*, Thorsons 1992) gives simple and easy-to follow guidelines on this important area of health care).
- To be really relaxed and able to cope with stress your diet needs to meet your requirements, while your intake of 'tasty toxins' and stimulants (coffee, tea, alcohol, tobacco, cola drinks, chocolate) needs to be as low as possible. There is more on this topic later in this chapter.
- Muscular release is the first step towards calming the mind (the mind *cannot* be calm if muscles are in tension). This might call for massage or stretching exercises.
- Your breathing needs to be full and free in order to be relaxed. Massage, exercise, stretching and breathing exercises can all help. Good breathing leads to better circulation and oxygenation, and

has specific calming effects on feelings of anxiety and 'being stressed out' – the body and mind cannot relax or cope well with stress if it is poorly supplied with vital oxygen and nutrients by a good blood supply, and this is as true for the scalp as for any other part of the body!

- Once you have achieved muscular release and full breathing, your mind needs to be able to stay still and focused and to release itself from the chatter of daily events and anxieties. This leads to a profound sense of being centred and at ease – and it shows to those around you as your ability to concentrate and remember details is boosted, and your whole being reflects calmness.

- Finally, once you have taken care of the muscular and breathing requirements, and your mind is still, you may wish to exercise it in 'creative visualization'. This can involve using the mind to travel to quiet, peaceful places, such as a sunlit meadow, a beach, riverside, or any other 'safe place'. You can also use it to visualize health improvements, such as the skin becoming clearer, mind and body more relaxed and healthy. There are many books and tapes to help guide you through this process, and I have included some in my book *The Stress Protection Plan* (Thorsons 1992).

To summarize: muscular release, full breathing, mental calm and guided imagery – these simple steps *in this sequence* can protect you from the worst effects of stress. They will also allow you to feel, function and look at your best with energy to spare, while enhancing your well-being and drastically improving your immune function.

CHAPTER FIVE

Food Allergy

An allergy is an altered (usually excessive) reaction to a substance, and varies from person to person. In most people, the substance produces no reaction; others may have a mild to moderate reaction; while some may react violently. This is different from a toxic reaction which would affect everyone more or less identically (cyanide kills everyone, but wheat sensitivity only upsets some people!).

An allergen (the substance to which the person is reacting) provokes the immune system, but only of the susceptible individual, to produce antibodies – defensive substances which are also produced in response to invading micro-organisms. It is the interaction between allergen and antibody that results in inflammatory defensive responses which, in the allergic person, will be excessive and produce symptoms, sometimes on the skin. Many instances have been found where seborrhoeic dermatitis relates directly to food allergy.

ARE YOUR SYMPTOMS DUE TO FOOD ALLERGY?

In the following questionnaire, scores are given (in brackets) for every answer. Work through these questions, then total up your score.

1 How often do you suffer from unnatural fatigue?
   • Daily (2)
   • Sometimes (1)
   • Never (0)

2 How often do you have weight fluctuations of 4 pounds (9 kilograms) or more in a day, with puffiness of the face, ankles or fingers?
   • Frequently (more than once a month) with or without severe puffiness (2)
   • Infrequently with or without slight puffiness (1)
   • Never (0)

3 How often do you find yourself sweating for no obvious reason (unless you have hot flushes)?
   • Frequently (several times a week or more) (2)
   • Infrequently (1)
   • Never (0)

4 How often does your heart race and/or pound strongly for no obvious reason?
   • Frequently (several times a week or more) (2)
   • Infrequently (1)
   • Never (0)

5 Have you any history of food intolerance causing any symptom?

- Yes (2)
- No (0)
6 Do you crave any of the following: bread, sugary foods, chocolate, milk, cheese, eggs, coffee or tea?
    - Yes (2)
    - No (0)
7 Do you suffer from *any* of the following: migraine, severe headaches irritable bowel syndrome, eczema, urticaria, depression, asthma or muscle aches?
    - Yes (2)
    - No (0)

The most anyone could score on this would be 14. If your score is 5 or higher, there is a likelihood that allergy is part of your symptom picture.

British expert Dr John Mansfield believes that there are 4 main factors at the root of food allergies:

1 Basic nutritional deficiencies (see chapter 6).
2 A repetitive, monotonous diet, where there is little variation in food families, and where the same pattern of eating is followed day after day for years on end. In some people, this can lead to them becoming 'sensitized' to particular foods.
3 Chemical adulteration of food.
4 Chronic intestinal yeast overgrowth (candidiasis).

He believes yeast infections such as *Candida* to be

the key to the upsurge in allergy which is now evident worldwide (J. Mansfield MD, *Arthritis – The Allergy Connection*, Thorsons 1990).

STONE-AGE DIET CONNECTION

Until humans became settled agricultural beings around 10,000 years ago, we lived as hunter-gatherers and ate hardly any dairy produce and virtually no grains. Research by Drs Boyd Eaton and Melvin Konner[1] describes the eating patterns of Stone-Age people. They consumed large amounts of animal protein and even larger amounts of fruits and plants but hardly any milk products or cereals.

It is the cereals and dairy products that form the highest percentage of human allergens worldwide. This has led to what is called the Primary Allergy Approach being developed in Sweden and now used throughout Europe[2]. This adopts a 'no cereals, no dairy products' diet as a first step in *all* allergies. Typically, many sensitivity/allergy problems other than the one being treated, vanish after a few weeks of this diet. In many cases, a gradual reintroduction of such foods is often possible on a rotation basis (the same food being consumed only every four to five days) once the person has become desensitized.

1. Eaton and Konner. 'Palaeolithic Nutrition', *New England Journal of Medicine*, January 1985
2. Based on the work of Ursulla Jonsson, Society Against Health Disorders, PO Box 38, S-87300 Bollstabruk, Sweden.

UNCOVERING YOUR ALLERGY

Michael Lesser MD of Berkeley California has compiled a 'timetable' which can often guide you to the meal that contained the offending food(s) or liquid(s) to which you may be reacting.[3]

Order of Appearances of Food-allergy Symptoms

Indigestion and heartburn	30 minutes
Headache	within 1 hour
Asthma or rhinitis (runny nose)	within 1 hour
Bloating of stomach and/or diarrhoea	3–4 hours
Rashes and hives	6–12 hours
Obvious weight gain through fluid retention	12–15 hours
Fits, confusion, mental disturbance	12–24 hours
Mouth ulcers, joint/muscle/ back aches/pain	48–96 hours

You can try to uncover your own allergies. This requires careful recording of what you eat and your symptoms. When you identify something that produces symptoms (such as those listed in the table above), you should eliminate this from the diet for some weeks to see what changes/ improvements occur without this food.

Alternatively, you can simply try to eliminate food families that have been medically identified as

3. Lesser, M. *Vitamin Therapy*, Parker House, California 1982

common allergens, such as dairy or grain products. Wait for a few weeks to see whether general and specific symptoms (such as dandruff) ease or vanish. If the offending substance is from the food family being tested, reintroducing the food family after a week or so would reproduce the symptoms (a worsening of dandruff, for example).

A good clue to possible personal allergens is found by looking at foods you eat every day, or foods you feel you could not manage without. When people are asked to think along these lines, they often mention bread or milk.

When there is a rapid rise or fall in pulse rate, from your normal resting level, there is evidence of exposure to a probable food or environmental allergen. Regular 'pulse' testing (before and after specific foods are eaten, for example) can be a way of applying careful detective work in uncovering culprit substances.

WHAT ABOUT BABIES?

Studies in Germany have shown that the delicate bowel flora of babies has altered over the past 25 years – for the worse. It is thought that this is largely due to the presence in almost all breast milk of substances such as dioxin and DDT which damage the intestinal flora (friendly bacteria) from birth. This is not to suggest that breast-feeding should be stopped – only that it is not as beneficial as it once was.[4]

The first colonies of 'friendly bacteria' in an infant are *Bifidobacteria infantis*. Levels of this in breast-fed babies are now found to be similar to the levels present in babies fed on formula (bottle) milk. This had led to a decline in immune-system efficiency; greater likelihood of infection; and increased levels of allergy, such as asthma and eczema (the incidences of which have trebled in ten years)[5]. Babies most likely to have cradle cap are the ones who have all or any of the following: lower immune function; increased infection patterns; increased allergic/sensitivity reactions.

One suggested remedy to the situation is supplementing babies' milk (whether breast or formula) with special 'infant' strains of these vital bacteria (as marketed in Britain and the United States as 'Lifestart' manufactured by Natren of California)[6].

No major changes in the diet of infants should be made without advice from a qualified expert – but it is certainly safe to eliminate dairy produce or grains if adequate care is taken over general nutritional balance.

4. Grutte and Muller Barthow. *Human Gastrointestinal Microflora*, J. Barth Verlag, Leipzig 1980
5. Report:'Asthma cases treble in ten years', *The Times*, London, 8 April 1992
6. For further information, see Chaitow, L. and Trenev, N. *Probiotics*, Thorsons 1991

A WORD OF CAUTION

If allergy appears to be part of your scalp or skin problem then the advice of a nutritional expert is called for. Self-help is certainly possible, but the complexity of achieving a balanced diet while at the same time removing major foods and/or whole 'food families' from the diet – leading perhaps to risks of deficiency – requires outside assistance.

CHAPTER SIX

Nutrition

The nutritional treatment of any condition can be divided into three essentially different but overlapping areas:

1 a sound nutritional base to maintain health and well-being
2 nutritional strategies to enhance overall immune function.
3 nutritional strategies that focus on specific symptoms and conditions

INDIVIDUALITY

There is no universal dietary prescription that will suit everyone. In each of the three categories listed above, we all start from different positions. We have varying histories both in terms of health and diet, as well as unique biochemical requirements which are inborn.

Some of the main differences are listed below:

- Some people will have eaten extremely well (in the real sense of the word) in the past (and present), while others will not, and may in fact be nutritionally deficient.
- Some people will be able to absorb nutrients from their food well while others will have badly impaired digestive and absorption capabilities (if, for example, they have yeast or allergy problems).
- During different phases of life there are quite distinct and exaggerated demands for particular nutrients. These include the growth period of childhood; spells of recovery from illness; during pregnancy; in advancing age; during phases of excessive physical activity. If these needs are not being met (and research shows that they commonly are not) then deficiency is a likely outcome.
- Some people will be overloaded with toxic debris from the past use of drugs, junk food and exposure to pollutants, while others will have no such burden.
- Because of what is known as 'biochemical individuality', some people will have specific nutrient requirements vastly different to those of others. Such differences are determined by genetic factors, over which the individual has no control.

GENERAL NUTRITIONAL GUIDELINES

Given the many possible variations in individual dietary needs, as listed above, it is feasible for this book to offer only *general* nutritional guidelines. The recommendations set out below are not meant as a prescription to be followed without expert guidance. Advice from a suitably qualified and licensed health-care professional is required to provide responsible *specific* nutritional guidelines.

Poorly balanced nutrition is one of the most important co-factors that influences the rate of progression of most common health problems. Without sound nutrition all other therapeutic efforts are bound to be less likely to succeed. A balanced wholefood diet is suggested (see below), usually accompanied by specific supplementation according to individual needs.

There are several possible reasons for disturbed nutritional status: poor choice of what is eaten; poor digestion/absorption of food, even if the diet is well balanced; problems in the way food is 'handled' by the body after it has been digested and absorbed because of disturbed transportation and utilization systems.

Listed below are just a few absolute directives that suit everyone:

1 Refined carbohydrates (sugar of any colour, white-flour products etc.) have been shown to depress immune function and to encourage metabolic mayhem. They should therefore be

avoided in anything but small amounts.

2 A diet high in saturated fats retards digestion.
   By increasing levels of cholesterol and certain
   fats, they also reduce the efficiency of specific
   aspects of the body's defence and repair
   mechanisms.

3 Animal fats (meat and dairy) should generally
   be avoided or reduced. However, oils from fish
   and many plants (especially those that have
   been cold-pressed, including olive, safflower,
   sunflower and linseed) are helpful in
   promoting immune function in general and
   skin function in particular. Avoid oils that have
   been hydrogenated (as in margarine), and
   beware of 'hidden fat' in biscuits and similar
   processed foods.

4 Alcohol and caffeine (coffee, tea, cola drinks,
   chocolate and cocoa) are known to affect
   immune efficiency negatively, and should be
   excluded as far as is possible from the diet.

5 Many additives are known to aggravate skin
   problems. One of the worst offenders is E102 –
   tartrazine.

6 If the digestive system is not easily able to
   handle raw foods such as vegetables, then an
   abundance of these nutrient-rich foods should
   be consumed lightly cooked (steamed or stir-
   fried, or in soups, stews etc.).

7 Assistance for the digestive system can be
   obtained via enzyme supplementation.

8 Protein intake needs to be kept at a good level

in order to supply adequate energy needs. Desirable sources of protein include low-fat live yoghurt, fish (especially of the cold-water varieties), free-range poultry and lean meat (game is best as it has lower fat levels than domesticated animal sources). Vegetarians should obtain protein from a daily combination of pulses and grains (unless there is allergy/sensitivity to them) as they combine to provide complete protein.

9 The ratio of proteins to carbohydrates and fats in the diet is important. Many health experts have emphasized that the ideal balance is 65 per cent complex carbohydrates (vegetables, fruits, pulses, grains); 15 per cent protein (fish, yoghurt, eggs, meat); and 20 per cent fat.

10 Choose 'dense' whole foods that are as unprocessed and additive-free as possible, and that require chewing.

11 Organic and fresh vegetables, fruits and proteins (fish/meat) should be chosen whenever possible.

12 Reduce or eliminate your intake of simple sugars and replace with complex carbohydrates (vegetables, whole grains, beans etc.) which are rich in nutrients (such as zinc).

13 Reduce polyunsaturated and saturated fats and oils – never fry food.

14 Use monounsaturated oils instead (such as olive oil) with special emphasis on omega–3 oils (fish and certain plant oils, such as linseed and borage).

15 Eat little and often throughout the day to
    optimize absorption of nutrients from food –
    five snack meals are better than one or two
    heavy meals.
16 Make sure fruits and vegetables are thoroughly
    clean and free of parasites and bacteria by
    peeling carefully or steaming lightly.
17 Eat a wide variety of foods to help avoid
    becoming sensitized to specific food families
    through frequent repetition.
18 Avoid chocolate, caffeine and alcohol
    completely.

Sample Menus

Here are a few suggestions for each meal. Choose
two or three selections for each meal. For drinks,
stick to herbal teas or spring water.

Breakfast

- Mixed seeds (sunflower, pumpkin, sesame,
  linseed) and grains (wheat or oat or millet or rice
  flakes or wholegrains). The seeds can be eaten
  whole or milled in a coffee grinder. They can be
  lightly oven-roasted or soaked overnight in a
  little water to soften them, and eaten with live
  low-fat yogurt and fresh fruit or on their own.
- Oatmeal (or millet) porridge plus fresh almonds
  or walnuts.
- Vegetable or fish soup with whole rice
  (unpolished) or wholegrain noodles.

- Live low-fat yoghurt or kefir.
- Sourdough rye or wheat bread or toast (depending on sensitivities/allergies) with olive oil or cottage cheese (low fat) or egg (see below).
- Enzyme-rich fruit, such as papaya.
- Tofu (bean curd) stir-fried with vegetables.
- Four or five eggs weekly (boiled, poached, scrambled).

Mid-morning and Mid-afternoon Snacks

Rice cakes or any of the items listed under 'breakfast'.

Lunch and Evening Meal

Unless a vegetarian diet has been chosen, at least one of these meals should contain an animal protein source such as fish, free-range poultry (avoiding skin) or game. If fish is chosen then a cold-water type such as herring, salmon, sardine, haddock, sole or cod should be eaten (avoid farmed fish as it may have antibiotic residues). Cook by boiling, steaming, grilling, casseroling, stir-frying or poaching, or use in a soup. Avoid frying or roasting as this alters the nature of any fat content. Protein should ideally be eaten with lightly cooked green vegetables and/or seaweed (available from Oriental or health-food shops). Seasoning should be by use of herbs (such as garlic) and spices, with as little salt as possible, or Oriental seasoning such as miso. If any oil is employed in cooking it should be virgin olive oil, which can also be used as a dressing.

The other main meal should be similar or could be based on a combination of pulses (chickpeas, mung beans, lentils, kidney or any other sort of bean) and grains (millet, brown rice, quinoa, amaranth, buckwheat etc.), either whole or as pasta/noodles). A soup, stew, roast or other combination of these ingredients (pulses/ grains) provides a first-class source of protein. Low-fat cheese (such as cottage) or tofu can also be eaten at this time. A variety of starchy vegetables (lightly cooked) such as carrot, beet, marrow, courgette and potato, as well as green vegetables, is also highly desirable, and there is abundant evidence of the health-enhancing value of brassica (cabbage, kale, broccoli). If digestion is sound, include raw salad as well. Desserts should be low-fat yoghurt (live) or enzyme-rich fruit (papaya, apple, pear). For vegetarians, the second main-meal option is ideal, and provides for many variations.

NUTRITIONAL SUPPLEMENTS

In addition to eating correctly it is usually necessary to supplement the diet with specific substances. These can help to normalize the biochemistry of the body which may have become deficient and unable to meet the demands made on it by the repair and defence mechanisms of the body. The reasons for such deficiencies are outlined below.

The term RDA refers to the recommended daily allowance of any particular vitamin or mineral to meet the essential needs of all 'healthy people'. The level is determined by panels of scientific advisers to governments, such as the Department of Health in Britain, and the FDA in the United States. The question is whether or not you are one of the 'healthy people' whose nutritional needs would be met by taking the RDA.

Even if it is accepted that this RDA level is accurate for healthy people (and this is strongly contested by many nutritionists who claim it to be inadequately low in most cases), the list of those who do not fit into the category of essentially healthy people is very wide. You might well be in one or more categories of people who require additional nutritional support in order to maintain health. Those who need extra support nutritionally include people:

- with very large or very small body sizes
- who live in hot climates or work in hot environments
- who are under stress at work
- who have wounds, burns or injuries
- who are taking prescribed medication (especially 'the Pill')
- who have digestive problems
- who are pregnant or breast-feeding
- who have unusual or unique metabolisms
- who have chronic illnesses

- who are involved in heavy regular exercise (training, aerobics etc.)
- who regularly consume alcohol *or* smoke (*or* live with a smoker)
- who regularly consume coffee
- who are involved in regular slimming diets
- who are past retirement age
- who are going through puberty
- who have infections
- who have too little or no exercise
- who are exposed to radiation (even by sun-bathing)
- who consume polluted water (i.e. most tap water)
- who are exposed to polluted air or pesticides
- who are under emotional stress

And if you do not fit into one of these categories there is another unhappy fact to absorb – that detailed surveys of almost all population groups (young children, school children, teenagers, young adults, middle-aged individuals in all socio-economic groups, and the elderly) regularly show that between 80 and 90 per cent fail to receive in their daily diet all the RDA of essential nutrients.

All of this comes on top of the established fact that, before we even start to consider the individual circumstances listed previously, we *all* begin with different nutritional requirements because of genetic programming. This is known medically as 'biochemical individuality', and it means that in the case of each of the nearly 50 different nutrients (vitamins, minerals etc.) which we need to survive in good health there will be variations in need from person to person – by up to 700 per cent in many instances.

Nutritionists and naturopaths find that in most cases of ill-health some dietary adjustment, and often supplementation, is needed to help recovery. In an ideal world we should get all our nutrients from our food. We do not – or at least this is the case for most of us – and so supplementation becomes a useful safety net, a health-insurance strategy, for health maintenance, for recovery from illness and for disease prevention.

It becomes a necessity when we are out of balance sufficiently to be manifesting symptoms of ill-health in a chronic way. Dandruff and skin rashes are evidence of such an imbalance.

Nutritional Support for Skin and Scalp Health

Pro-vitamin A (Betacarotene)

Betacarotene is basically non-toxic (unlike vitamin A itself, which should be taken only under expert guidance in anything but small amounts because it is fat soluble and potentially toxic). A daily dose of 15,000–30,000 iu of beta carotene is suggested. If vitamin A itself is being taken, a daily dose of no more than 10,000 iu is recommended.

B-complex

One slow-release B-complex capsule is commonly suggested to be taken daily. This should be formulated to a high potency (50–100 mg of each of the major B vitamins). Please note that yeast-free sources of B vitamins are recommended by many experts to avoid possible aggravation of sensitivities resulting from yeast infections such as *Candida albicans*.

Pantothenic Acid (Vitamin B_5)

The recommended dosage is 200–300 mg daily.

Pyridoxine (Vitamin B_6)

Vitamin B6 is involved in many aspects of immune function and is commonly deficient. A dose of 100 mg daily, taken at a different meal to that at which you take B complex, is suggested.

Inositol

100 mg daily.

Biotin

A B-vitamin usually produced by a healthy bowel flora, biotin becomes deficient as a result of damage to the 'friendly bacteria' of the intestines. When deficient, it is thought to increase virulence of yeast overgrowth (*Candida*), a common co-factor infection in people whose immune system is vulnerable. Biotin is very important in treatment of seborrhoeic dermatitis and dandruff, and a dose of 2 mg daily is suggested for adults, and 500 mcg to 1 mg daily for children.

Selenium and Vitamin E

A mineral symbiotic with vitamin E, selenium is also the main ingredient of most anti-dandruff shampoos ('Selsun' and others). A suggested daily adult dosage is 400 iu of vitamin E and 200 mcg of selenium.

Vitamin C (Ascorbic Acid)

At least 1 gram daily, preferably 3, should be taken regularly with meals.

Zinc

Nutritional experts have suggested that practically all people with skin problems such as dandruff and SD are deficient in zinc. Since nearly 100 important enzymes depend upon adequate presence of zinc, and many of these are involved in immune function, zinc supplementation is important. A daily dosage of 30–50 mg is usual. Other symptoms which are common when zinc is deficient include:

- skin lesions (ulceration, thickening, dryness)
- loss of hair
- loss of appetite
- reduced sense of smell
- lethargy
- increased susceptibility to infection

Essential Fatty Acids

Supplementation with essential fatty acids is extremely helpful in normalizing skin and scalp problems. Omega 3 and Omega 6 fatty acids are 'essential', which means that humans cannot manufacture them and have to have a dietary intake. Anyone with skin or scalp problems should supplement the diet with a good source of oils containing linoleic acid, as well as gamma linolenic acid, derived from the evening primrose plant, blackcurrent seeds, borage (herb) or linseed, as well as from fish oils (which provides eicosapentenoic acid – EPA). The dosage should be between 1–3 grams daily. Vegetarians should rely on flaxseed oil as the body can usually transform the form of EFA found in this to the form found in fish. For non-vegetarians, however, the fish oil source is the easiest way.

Probiotics – 'Friendly Bacteria'

Almost every person with chronic skin problems, including dandruff, has some degree of compromised internal ecology affecting their bowel flora. When the flora are healthy they help detoxify the bowel, manufacture B-vitamins and keep yeasts and undesirable bacteria in check. The flora is easily damaged by antibiotics, steroid drugs, unbalanced diet and stress.

Supplementation of *L. acidophilus* and *Bifidobacteria* (see page 23) is suggested for some months to help normalize the intestinal ecology.

Silica

This derives from the horsetail herb, and is useful for improving hair quality.

Multivitamin/mineral Supplements

As an 'insurance' against deficiency, a soundly constructed multivitamin/mineral supplement is a useful option in order to provide an underlying source of nutrients.

THE VALUE OF NUTRITION

The eating of a sound, balanced, nutritious diet is probably the single most important factor over which most people have control – if economic circumstances allow. This does not have to be excessively expensive, and indeed there is evidence that processed, 'junk' food is more expensive, both financially and in health terms.

Without becoming obsessive, it is fair to say that application of nutritional exellence in modern life has a greater impact on the level of health, the frequency of illness and the likelihood of a long life than any other factor over which we have control – and minor symptoms such as dandruff are a good indicator of how well you are doing in achieving this ideal.

CHAPTER SEVEN

Toxicity

Your skin is a powerful and vital organ. It is virtually a 'second lung' through which your body eliminates a great deal of waste material – when it is healthy, that is. Your circulatory system carries metabolic wastes (produced normally as by-products of natural body functions) to the skin along tiny capillaries to be excreted through the pores.

The outer surface of the skin is made up of 'dead' cells which you shed all the time. When, however, these dead skin cells become covered with microscopic particles of dirt and oils (which you produce yourself), the body's easy elimination processes through the pores can be blocked or slowed. Such blockages lead to blemishes, pimples and blackheads and, if the conditions are right, to seborrhoeic dermatitis (and dandruff).

A number of simple detoxification procedures are described below. These can be used to normalize skin function, improving the tone, eliminating toxins and mobilizing fatty deposits lying below the skin surface (cellulite).

BENEFITS OF DETOXIFYING

Your overall health can also benefit from these detoxification methods. When your skin is working efficiently, your level of toxicity drops, putting less strain on other organs of elimination, such as the liver, kidneys, bowels and lungs. As toxic deposits are removed from the system, not only should you 'feel' better, but you will also have more energy and greater vitality.

And, of course, there is the final result of detoxifying (which is probably your main objective since you are reading this book) – firmer and clearer skin with a better colour and surface condition, and the disappearance of dandruff.

WHERE DO TOXINS COME FROM?

Most people today have been exposed to, and will have absorbed, toxic materials. These can be from the environment (food, air and water), from medication and drugs, and from toxic habits (such as smoking). The residual toxins in the body are poisonous burdens which aggravate tissues and organs. They sometimes cause health problems, especially in the skin which, being a major route for toxic elimination, is often affected by toxicity.

Before deciding to detoxify, get advice from a health professional to help you select the degree of intensity with which you should apply the various methods available, some of which are described below. If you are robust and vital, a more vigorous programme will be needed than if you are unwell and somewhat fragile in your health.

I have set out a series of tests and questionnaires in my book *Clear Body Clear Mind* (Thorsons, 1990) which can help you identify your current level of toxicity. The following is a shortened version which will help you to know whether or not you need to detoxify.

CLUES TO TOXICITY

One strong indication that you may need to detoxify is the more-or-less constant presence of particular symptoms. If symptoms fluctuate, vary from day to day or week to week, they are probably allergic in origin; if they are cyclical – predictably so – then they are probably hormonal or seasonally allergic; whereas if they are constant they may be toxic in origin.

Questionnaire

1 Have you or do you come into regular close proximity with chemicals, heavy metals,

vinyl, cleaning materials or industrial by-products?

2 Do you live or work in an industrial area, a smog-laden environment or close (less than half a mile) to heavy traffic routes?

3 Is your work place or home air-conditioned, double-glazed or centrally heated?

4 Are the walls of your work place or home foam-insulated?

5 Have you more than four mercury amalgam fillings in your teeth, or do you work in or near a dental surgery?

6 Have you or your colleagues at work ever complained that the building is subject to 'sick building syndrome'?

7 Are your water pipes at home or work made of lead or copper, and whether or not the answer to this is 'yes', do you drink tap water – even in tea?

8 Are you in a soft-water area ?

9 In your hobbies or at work do you use sprays, varnishes, paints, glue, sanding or polishing equipment, or do you inhale brick powder, wood dust or other fumes?

10 Do you have contact in work or hobby (gardening) with herbicides, pesticides or artificial fertilizers?

11 Do you service or maintain your own car – or do that sort of work for a living ?

12 Do you swim in chlorinated water once a week or more?

13 Do you travel by air on average more than 300 miles (500 km) weekly; or do you travel by air more than twice a year? Do you travel by city-based public transport four or more times weekly; or are you active outdoors in a city for more than 30 minutes four times a week?

14 Do you paint (pictures or walls!) for a hobby or a living?

Any 'yes' answers mean that you have some toxic exposure – and depending on the efficiency of your organs of detoxification (liver, kidneys, skin) you will handle this more or less adequately. The more 'yes' answers there are, the greater the toxic burden – and the greater the chances of your needing to detoxify.

A DETOXIFICATION PROGRAMME

Whether your general health is adequate for you to undertake rapid and active detoxification, or whether it would be better to string the process out and to do the job slowly is a matter for the judgement of a qualified health professional such as a naturopath. Whichever speed and intensity is more appropriate, the ingredients of the detox program are the same – it is only the speed and strength of what is done that needs to be modified according to your individual needs.

The following detox program is safe for almost everyone – but do check with your health adviser first. *If you are a recovering drug user or alcoholic, or if you have an eating disorder or are a diabetic, then certainly **do not** apply these methods without asking professional advice first.*

Priority number one in detoxification is dietary, and the following methods are effective. Over *almost every weekend* for a few months (and thereafter once a month at least) choose between the following:

A Short, Water-only Fast

This fast lasts for 24 to 36 hours, and should be conducted over a weekend. You can start on Friday evening and end on Saturday evening, or just fast all day Saturday so that work schedules are not interfered with. Make sure that no less than 4, and no more than 8, pints of bottled water are consumed during the day (2–4.5 litres). On the Sunday, have a raw-food day, eating only fruit and salad, which should be chewed well, and drinking as much water as you like (up to the amount already mentioned).

A Full-weekend Fast

To begin with, this fast should be followed each weekend or at least three a month. Starting on Friday night and going through to Sunday evening, follow a 'monodiet'. This means choosing a single food from the following:

- Any type of fruit. Your choice could be grapes, apples, pears (best choice if an allergy history exists) or papaya (ideal if digestive problems exist). Eat up to 3 pounds (1.5 kg) daily.
- Brown rice, buckwheat, millet or potatoes (skin and all) – boiled and eaten whenever desired, and made palatable by adding a little lemon juice and olive oil. You may eat up to a pound (dry weight) of any of the grains (0.5 kg), or 3 pounds (1.5 kg) of potatoes daily over the weekend.

Whichever type of weekend detox you choose, make sure you rest and keep warm, and that you have no engagements or dates. This is a time to allow all available energy to focus on the repairing and cleansing processes of detoxification.

What to Expect

In the early days (first few weekends) you could develop a headache and furred tongue – this is fine. It will slowly get less obvious as detoxification progresses. Take nothing to stop the headache, and rest as much as you can.

As the weeks pass, your skin should become clearer (it may get a bit spotty for a while), your eyes clearer, brain sharper and digestion more efficient. Your energy levels should rise and you should regain a feeling of youthful clarity you had forgotten.

When the tongue no longer becomes furred and headaches no longer appear you can begin to spread these intensive detox weekends apart – three a month and then two a month, and then maintenance fasts once a month.

What to Eat Between Fasts

In between these weekend detoxification intensives, a milder midweek programme of gentle detoxification could involve the following pattern (assuming that you are not already following a special diet, such as the anti-yeast one described in chapter 3).

Breakfast
- Fresh fruit (raw or lightly cooked – no sweetening) and live yoghurt
- *or* home-made muesli (seeds and nuts and grains) and live yoghurt
- *or* cooked grains and yoghurt (buckwheat, millet, linseed, barley, rice etc.).
- Drink herbal tea (linden blossom, chamomile, mint, sage, lemon verbena) or hot water and lemon.

Lunch/supper
- One of these meals should be a raw salad with jacket potato or brown rice and either bean curd

(tofu), low-fat cheese or nuts/seeds.

- If raw food is a problem, choose a stir-fried vegetable/tofu meal or steamed vegetables eaten with potato or rice together with low fat cheese or nuts and seeds.
- The other main meal should be a choice between fish, chicken, game or vegetarian savoury (pulse/grain combination) and vegetables lightly steamed, baked or stir-fried.
- For desserts, choose lightly stewed fruit (add apple or lemon juice, not sugar), or live natural yoghurt.

Remember to season food with garlic and herbs, avoiding salt as much as possible. Eat slowly, chew well, do not drink with meals, and consume at least two pints of liquid daily between meals.

The periods between fasting weekends can also include a few 'naughty but nice' tasty toxins from time to time – making social life a bit more relaxed. By this time your internal detox system should be able to cope with such indiscretions.

SUPPLEMENTS FOR DETOX SUPPORT

Take one high-potency multivitamin/mineral capsule daily; 1 gram of vitamin C; 400 iu of vitamin E; and three garlic capsules with meals. Also take a daily acidophilus supplement for bowel detox support (the 'Natren' brand is recommended, see chapter 3 for details).

Vitamin C and E are especially important if chemical toxicity is involved. This is because they act as antioxidants (as does garlic), 'switching off' dangerous free-radical molecule activity which damages tissues.

CHAPTER EIGHT

Treatments for Scalp and Skin Health

The skin has some amazing qualities. Although it serves as a protective envelope, it will also allow substances to pass through it in both directions – to eliminate wastes and to let nutrients and herbal essences in. We can use this knowledge when treating scalp and skin problems.

This chapter looks at ways in which we can treat the skin in order to improve dandruff and related problems. It is essential to bear in mind, however, that the systemic methods – using nutrition and supplementation for example – which were described in previous chapters should be seen to be the foundations underpinning anything you do on a local level.

Remember that most SD skin conditions on the face, behind the ears and on the neck start on the scalp. If you clear the dandruff the other skin problems will almost certainly vanish – especially if you are dealing with systemic needs as well.

There are several different methods you can use

to enhance general skin function, and specifically that of the scalp. A few methods should be used regularly, others now and then, when you feel like it or when they are indicated by a need to help detoxification.

Before we look at specific advice for dealing with seborrhoeic dermatitis and dandruff, some basic guidelines follow which could save you from self-inflicted damage to your scalp and crowning glory.

FACTS ABOUT THE SCALP AND HAIR

- It is perfectly normal to lose a number of hairs (between 50 and 80 daily) throughout life, so do not worry about this small amount of hair loss. Most of it will grow back healthily.
- Hair and scalp care involves just the same factors as any other part of the body – and this demands that you keep both the scalp and hair well nourished and in a hygienic state, with as little destructive exposure to chemicals and harsh conditions (such as heat) as possible.
- A diet that nourishes you will also nourish your scalp and hair. Protein deficiency will seriously weaken the strength of hair and lead to actual hair loss as well as resulting in a less than healthy scalp. You are most likely to have such a deficiency when you are ill, or when following a specialized or restricted eating pattern for any reason, especially during and

following periods of stringent dieting.

- Be aware that use of particular medications (such as 'the Pill', anticoagulants and, in particular, certain anti-cancer drugs) can have negative effects on hair and scalp status, as can pregnancy, menopause and periods of hormonal imbalance.

- Hair loss following pregnancy is common – but if nutrition is sound this should grow back within a few months. A similar pattern of hair loss may follow after stopping taking the Pill – again the reason is largely hormonal, and if diet is sound hair growth should normalize within a few months as hormonal balance is restored.

- Conditions such as diabetes, iron deficiency anaemia and any illness involving the endocrine glands (such as thyroid imbalances) or where circulation is seriously impaired, will usually produce changes in hair quality. In a hypothyroid condition, where there is low production of the thyroid hormones, the hair of the outer third of the eyebrows tends to fall out – an easy clue to observe.

NUTRITION AND SCALP HEALTH

A balanced intake of vitamins and minerals is essential for health of scalp and hair. The following nutrients, in particular, have been found helpful:

- Essential fatty acids (omega 6) from oils such as

those found in evening primrose, borage and flaxseed (500–1,000 mg daily).

- Essential fatty acids (omega 3) such as those found in fish oils (1,000 mg daily). Vegetarians should rely on flaxseed oil as the body can usually change the form of EFA found in this to the form found in fish. For non-vegetarians, fish oil is the best option.
- A good potency vitamin B-complex (one daily with food).
- Additional individual B vitamins that can help scalp and hair status include B5 (pantothenic acid) – 200–300 mg daily; B6 (pyridoxine) – 200 mg daily; B3 (niacin) – 100 mg daily; inositol – 100 mg daily. These vitamins should be taken at a different time from the B-complex.
- Vitamin E, which is especially useful for scalp health (200–400 iu daily).
- Zinc, which is most important for helping to heal scalp damage and to promote hair growth (100 mg daily).
- Coenzyme Q10, a powerful (but expensive) aid to normalizing poor circulation to the scalp and to its regeneration (50 mg daily).
- Silica, which derives from the horsetail herb, is useful for improving hair quality.
- For women, taking 600 iu of vitamin E and 1 gram of vitamin C daily can lower levels of the male hormone testosterone and enhance oestrogen levels. This is useful around the menopause if there is associated hair loss.

Herbs

- Sage can be used as a hair tonic. Make an infusion of this herb (in the way in which you make tea) and rinse the hair with it after shampooing.
- Apple cider vinegar can also be used as a tonic after shampooing.
- Millet extracts are useful for hair and scalp care. A number of Swiss products are available through specialized shops).

HOW TO AVOID DAMAGE

- Harsh, vigorous, prolonged, frequent or excessive brushing; vigorous massage or combing; and the use of undesirable chemicals in washing or grooming are all damaging to the hair and scalp and should be avoided unless they are part of a treatment protocol.
- Unless hair is oily, daily shampooing is undesirable (except when specifically prescribed as a treatment), as is use of bleach and colouring agents.
- Brushing or combing hair when it is wet is likely to cause more damage than when it is dry – and should therefore be avoided.
- Brushes should not be excessively hard-bristled, and natural ones are better than those made of synthetic materials.
- When using a blow-dryer, keep it warm, not hot, and stop as soon as you can – natural

drying is far better for the scalp and hair.

- Excessive pull on the hair damages the roots, causes split ends and breaks in the shaft of the hair – so backcombing and plaiting and any style (bun, plait, ponytail etc.) which calls for a lot of mechanical tension on the hair is undesirable. These styles can be achieved without the pull being excessive and this should not cause damage.
- Chemicals such as bleach or those found in most swimming pools (and in tap water to a lesser degree) are oxidizing agents – as is sunshine – and all will cause free-radical damage which is hard to reverse.
- Use medicated shampoos only if you need to.
- Tightly rolling washed hair before drying causes much the same damage as tight buns and braiding. Roll the hair loosely.
- Hot rollers that actually touch the scalp are likely to produce skin damage in time – take great care to avoid chemicals, heat and mechanical stress.
- Choose conditioners and shampoos carefully – go for the most natural (such as those meant for dry hair). These are often the least expensive.

DANDRUFF SHAMPOOS, LOTIONS AND TONICS

Dr Goodman ('the skin doctor') and other experts

have suggested guidelines for the use of local treatments – applying shampoos and other preparations to the hair and scalp. Most of these experts believe that the mainstay of successful dandruff treatment is 'proper' shampooing and scalp hygiene. The key guidelines are as follows:

- Use an appropriate shampoo daily – or at least three times a week.
- Only a mild, non-medicated shampoo is required if the seborrhoeic dermatitis (dandruff) is mild.
- If the condition is more severe, use a stronger, anti-dandruff (medicated) shampoo at least once a week in addition to the other shampooing.
- In cases of severe dandruff problems local medication or herbal application is probably also called for.
- If medicated shampoos are being used to treat severe and long-standing dandruff, at least two, and ideally three, different types should be employed. This prevents 'resistance' developing because of the persistent use of just one type.

There are different forms of medicated shampoo – and in any given case one or two will be more suitable than others. Only trial and error will show which is right for you. If there is a yeast problem then the selenium-based ones will act best. The different types include:

- Zinc Pyrithione (including 'Head and Shoulders' and 'Danex').
- Selenium sulfide (including 'Selsun' and 'Lenium').
- Sulfur/Salicylic acid (including 'Ionil' and 'Sebulex').
- Parachlorometaxylenol (including 'Metasep').
- Tar-based shampoos (including 'Denorrex' and 'Sebutone') – all of which can stain light-coloured (blond, grey, bleached) hair.
- Shampoos containing nutrients or herbs which try to heal the scalp less aggressively by a more 'natural' route.

In addition to regular shampooing with a variety of medicated and herbal substances, local treatment using 'tonics' or lotions can be extremely useful in encouraging improved circulation, ridding the scalp surface of dead skin and reducing itching. Again, there are many products to choose from, ranging from gentle millet-based products to those deriving from peat or clay or from herbs such as nettles and sage. A selection of these is listed on page 83, all of which should be available from good health stores and pharmacies.

Also available are medicated scalp dressings based on the same chemicals used in medicated shampoos. These include tar, sulphur and, for the most serious cases of scalp seborrhoea, hydrocortisone-based lotions, creams and gels (these are suitable for short-term use only).

There is also a wide range of products which are neither plain shampoos nor medicated products, but based on naturally occurring chemicals and herbs. These include the excellent range of products from Austria's Neydharting Moor, from Switzerland (millet extracts), Israel (Dead Sea products) and France (clay products), all of which have shown success in treating skin and scalp problems. In some cases, these treatments have proved more successful than standard medical approaches (psoriasis success by Dead Sea products is famous worldwide). Some of these approaches are listed on pages 76–8.

Should You Use Medicated Products?

This must be a very personal choice. Most of these products are reasonably harmless and safe if used *precisely* as the manufacturers suggest. None of them, however, will 'cure' dandruff unless systemic methods are also used (see chapters 2–7). If systemic methods are used then herbal methods are likely to be just as successful as medicated methods of scalp care – but will take a good deal longer to work. The main advantage of using regular medicated shampoos and lotions is their speed of action.

The downside of using medicated shampoos is that they may produce resistance to their effectiveness, especially if only one type is being used. They are also more likely to produce reactions in people with extreme sensitivity/allergy problems.

CHOOSING AND APPLYING TREATMENTS

Only you can decide which type of dandruff treatment is best for you, and the variety of choices available is enormous. I suggest that, after commencing the systemic methods appropriate for your needs, you experiment with a variety of the medicated shampoos and lotions for several weeks each, and that you also use some of the herbal approaches as described on pages 79–81 (unless you have a philosophical reason for avoiding them, such as a concern to avoid products tested on animals – as most medicated shampoos are – or if you prefer 'natural' to chemical products).

Your selection of what to use – depending upon what is available and how much it all costs – should not influence how often you apply these methods – frequency is almost as important as the substances used. As you will see later, there are ways of making your own inexpensive hair tonics and rinses – but not shampoos.

If you are regularly applying adequate local care, following the methods described on pages 74–5, and are also paying attention to systemic factors (nutrition, stress reduction and general skin treatments) you should see rapid progress towards a healthy scalp.

For the first few weeks of treatment, however, hair may become dry and brittle. In some instances, the rate of normal hair loss may be accelerated. This will normalize and correct itself, especially if you follow the advice given below regarding care and attention following shampooing. Avoid using hot blow-dryers more than once a week, allowing drying to be natural whenever practical.

You may also experience an apparent increase in your dandruff during the first weeks of your campaign. This, too, is normal as the concentrated effort will be helping you shed more loose flakes. After a short time, this tendency will settle down.

Shampooing Method

It is important to be aware of the precise way in which you should shampoo and care for your scalp and hair. The following guidelines will help.

- Shampoo at least three times weekly, but daily if possible at first (several weeks).
- If the condition is severe, use a medicated shampoo at least once a week, with other non-medicated (herbal or standard shampoos) at other times.
- Each time you shampoo use a different product from the last time. Rotating two or three shampoos is particularly important if you are using medicated versions so that you reduce the chances of resistance to their effectiveness developing.

- Work the shampoo sufficiently to build up a lather. If this does not form the first time then rinse and shampoo again. Once the lather is present leave it in place for between five and ten minutes.
- If you find it difficult to get a lather the reason may be that your hair is too long or too oily. Consider having a shorter style for a while and/or perhaps apply an additional (third) lathering to ensure that this substance can be left in place long enough to do its work – perhaps under a towel while you wait.
- While shampooing/lathering use vigorous fingertip contact on the entire scalp (or use a rubber, *not* plastic, scrubbing device with lots of tiny projections) to massage the scalp thoroughly but gently and loosen dead skin.
- Before applying conditioner, or at another time of day, use a scalp tonic or lotion combined with more massage of the scalp.
- After lathering, rinse and apply a conditioner if you wish (which helps to prevent hair from becoming stressed).

Applying Tonics and Lotions

It is no use whatever sprinkling a scalp lotion onto your hair and rubbing hopefully for a while! To dress the scalp it is necessary to get the lotion onto the skin of the head itself. To achieve this, dampen the hair and make a parting as far to one side of the head as you can. Then apply a few drops of the lotion along that parting.

Make another parting a quarter of an inch closer to the centre, and again apply lotion to the skin down that parting. Proceed right across the head as far as you can until you have applied lotion – drop by drop – to the entire head. Massage the scalp with your fingertips for at least two minutes, then comb or brush the hair.

ADDITIONAL METHODS

Use these methods in between or after your regular shampooing, as described earlier, not instead of it.

Dead Sea Products

These contain a remarkable array of minerals and naturally occurring chemicals such as sulphur, and have an impressive track record of success in treating skin conditions such as SD, dandruff, eczema and especially psoriasis. The protocol recommended by the importers of Dead Sea products for dandruff care is as follows:

- For mild dandruff wash the hair every day for a week using Dead Sea shampoo for dry hair (DSD) ensuring that lather remains on the scalp for at least two minutes before washing off.
- As the condition improves reduce to twice-weekly maintenance treatments.

- For severe dandruff massage the scalp with shampoo straight from the bottle, and allow it to remain in place for not less than ten minutes before shampooing off.

These methods are effective but require patience. Although they take time to work, the effects tend to be long-lasting (see also Chapter 9).

Neydharting Moor Shampoo

This dandruff treatment is recommended by many nutritionists and herbalists who suggest following it with the application of Neydharting hair tonic while the hair is still wet. These products contain literally thousands of chemicals derived from plants which have formed the moor over the past 20,000 years. Extensive research has validated the claims made for these products.

Schuppexin Tonic

This Swiss millet-based product is manufactured by Haar Sana and contains chamomile, gentian, other Alpine herbs and millet extract. It is suggested that this be massaged daily into the scalp until the condition normalizes. Shampooing should involve use of Millet shampoo (also by Haar Sana), which contains coconut oil. The rich lather should be left in place for several minutes before rinsing – and the manufacturers claim no conditioner is needed after its use.

Corpore Sana

From Italy come products which include Hop and Thyme shampoo for dandruff treatment, and Nettle and Witch Hazel shampoo for seborrhoeic problems – ideal if hair is oily. These should be used according to the guidelines given for Schuppexin.

Aromatherapy and Other Oils

The next five suggestions can be messy!

1) Essential oils of cedarwood, lavender and rosemary can be blended to make an aromatherapy treatment. Add ten drops of each oil to a quarter of a cup of carrier oil (such as coconut). Massage this into the scalp and leave on overnight (wear a turban, towel or at least use old pillowcases). Wash off in the morning using a non-medicated shampoo, and then use a natural tonic as suggested below.

2) If there is a yeast problem (see Chapter 3) add ten drops of tea tree oil and ten drops of jojoba oil to a sunflower or almond-oil carrier (a quarter of a cupful). Massage into the scalp at night, for three nights running once a fortnight, until the problem is under control. In the morning use a medicated selenium-based shampoo to wash the hair and scalp.

3) Vitamin E oil (in its bottled or capsule form) is recommended by many nutritionists. The oil should be applied to the scalp nightly for at

least three weeks. During the day, apply a hair tonic made from an infusion of one ounce (28 grams) each of rosemary, nettle and sage infused in 2 pints (1 litre) of water for 24 hours.

4) Some old texts suggest using castor oil instead of Vitamin E oil (see Chapter 9 for its use in treating psoriasis of the scalp).

5) As part of an anti-dandruff campaign which also includes nutritional methods, Drs Stephen Davies and Alan Stewart recommend another messy but effective local treatment in which cold-pressed linseed oil is applied to the scalp at night (again, take precautions to protect your bed linen). In the morning this should be washed off with an anti-dandruff shampoo (containing selenium if possible). This can be used as an anti-fungal, anti-dandruff approach three times weekly.

Herbal Treatments

Herbalist David Hoffman suggests that you rinse your hair and scalp regularly using a strong infusion of nettles, sage and rosemary. His other suggestions include drinking nettle tea several times daily, and taking 500 mg of oil evening primrose three times a day. Use the infusion after a shampoo (regular not medicated), accompanied by a gentle but thorough massage of the scalp. Then wrap your hair in a damp towel for at least five minutes.

Another (traditional) method of treatment is to pour warm apple cider vinegar over the scalp, and to wrap the head swiftly with a towel, leaving it in place for an hour before washing with a nettle shampoo.

Infusion for Dry Skin or Scalp

You will need half an ounce (14 grams) each of at least four of the following:

- chamomile
- rose petals
- rosemary
- violets (leaf or flower or both)
- comfrey (leaf or root or both)
- acacia flowers

Place in a saucepan with 4½–5 pints (2.5–3 litres) of water. Bring to the boil and allow to simmer for 15 minutes. Strain and place fluid in the bath to treat general skin dryness, or use locally (a cup or two at a time) to soak the scalp and hair thoroughly, ideally after washing with an unmedicated shampoo. Wrap the hair in a damp towel for at least five minutes before drying.

Infusion for Oily Skin or Hair

You will need half an ounce (14 grams) each of at least four of the following:

- witch-hazel bark
- lemon peel

- raspberry leaf
- lemon grass
- peppermint
- orange flowers or peel
- chamomile

Place in a saucepan with 4½–5 pints (2.5–3 litres) of water. Bring to the boil and allow to simmer for 15 minutes. Strain and place fluid in the bath to treat general skin oiliness, or use locally (a cup or two at a time) to soak the scalp and hair thoroughly, ideally after washing with an unmedicated shampoo. Wrap the hair in a damp towel for at least five minutes before drying.

Face and Scalp Sauna

This treatment is ideal for general cleansing. You can buy inexpensive equipment that will allow steam to be brought to your face or head for cosmetic and therapeutic purposes. Far cheaper, however, is the use of a bowl and a towel and/or umbrella. For deep cleansing of the pores of the scalp and face, this home sauna is a super-efficient method. The method is described below.

For extra benefit, use a variety of essential oils or herbs. Choose from:

- rose petals
- lavender
- chamomile flowers
- elder blossom

- acacia
- mint
- sage
- chickweed
- comfrey leaf and/or root
- raspberry leaf
- strawberry leaf
- slippery elm bark

Add half an ounce (14 grams) of each of at least four of the herbs to 3½ pints (2 litres) of water in a saucepan. Bring to the boil and allow to simmer for two to three minutes. Remove from the heat and leave to cool for a minute or so, then pour the liquid into a large bowl.

Place a towel over your entire head so that it drapes over your face and the bowl, and so that your face (eyes closed) and head/scalp are in direct contact with the rising herb-laden steam. Stay in the steam for at least five, ideally ten minutes, and then splash the face and scalp with cold water. Pat dry, then apply a scalp tonic (see below). Do this at least once a week on a day when you are not shampooing the hair.

Normal or Dry Skin or Scalp

Use the sauna method as outlined above, but this time use an ounce (28 grams) each of peppermint and chamomile and 2 ounces (14 grams) of lemon grass.

Oily Skin or Scalp

Use the same sauna method as outlined above, but this time use an ounce (28 grams) each of basil, comfrey root and rosemary.

Aromatherapy Sauna

This treatment is for dry, normal and mature skin. Bring to the boil 1¾ pints (1 litre) of water, and allow it to cool for two minutes. Pour the water into a bowl and add to it four drops each of geranium and lavender oil, and two drops of patchouli. Cover your entire head and bowl with a towel and let the vapours treat your skin and scalp for five minutes or so. Finish with a cold splash before drying under a towel and then use a scalp tonic (see below).

For oily skin or scalp use the previous method, but this time add four drops each of lemon essence, cypress and juniper.

Scalp and Skin Tonics

After any local treatment that involves steaming, always use a toner, tonic or freshener on facial or head skin. If there is a tendency to dryness, a natural moisturizer should be used as well. On the scalp use one of the following after a local sauna:

- millet tonic
- nettle tonic
- Dead Sea scalp treatment
- moor hair tonic

GENERAL SKIN DETOXIFICATION AND ENHANCEMENT

These methods will *indirectly* assist in resolution of dandruff, but most are not specifically aimed at this condition.

Skin-brushing (Dry Method)

This is best done 'dry' before you wash, shower or bathe, and it need take only a few minutes (five at most). Once you decide to start using skin-brushing to improve your skin and health you should also make up your mind that it will become a daily routine. It makes you feel (and look) so good that soon you will feel as lost without it as you would if you forgot to brush your teeth!

Equip yourself with a bath-mitt, loofah or a natural bristle body-brush. Make sure the room is warm and there are no draughts. You need to be fully unclothed to do this job effectively. Skin-brushing can be done standing, but sitting on a stool allows you to deal with backs of legs and other 'difficult' parts more efficiently, without having to perform contortions.

You should start by brushing gently. At first you can expect a 'red reaction', which shows that your circulation is responding to the stimulation you are giving it. The action of brushing needs to be circular, 'creeping' and firm, but not irritating. The circular motion helps you avoid rubbing over one area too much (once or twice over any part of the skin is adequate at first), and the 'creeping' has the same effect. This simply means that, without lifting the brush, you gradually slide towards the next part of the skin which is due to receive attention.

Be particularly gentle with the skin on the backs of legs and arms, as well as your back, abdomen and chest, as these areas may be more sensitive and tender. Avoid breast tissue and be very careful with the inner thighs. After a week or so of repetitive skin-brushing, the skin that was tender will be less so, and you can slowly increase the pressure and vigour of your brushing.

If there are bits of your back you cannot reach, rub your back briskly with a dry towel. It will not be as effective as a brush, mitt or loofah but will be better than no friction at all.

Skin-brushing (Wet Method)

This method is basically the same as the dry one, except that you start by taking a shower or a bath. Before drying yourself, perform the process as described for dry brushing but moisten the brush, mitt or loofah as well. Shower afterwards, ideally finishing with water around body temperature or cooler.

The Salt Glow

This is a wonderful skin tonic and detoxification

method. Basically a skin-friction treatment using wet, coarse (sea) salt or Epsom salts, the Salt Glow is particularly beneficial for people who have difficulty sweating or who have poor circulation to their hands and/or feet. It is also useful for people prone to rheumatic aches and pains. If you can, get someone else to adminster the Salt Glow to you, as self-treatment cannot reach all parts of your body – just imagine trying to rub effectively *all* of your back yourself!

Unlike the skin-brushing method which is suggested as a daily routine, the Salt Glow is an occasional treatment – once a week at most if you have difficulty sweating, and once a month or so for general detoxification purposes.

You will need a bowl and at least 6 ounces (170 grams) of coarse salt or Epsom salts. Sit on a stool in the bath or shower and add water to the salt in the bowl to moisten it – just enough to make the salt grains stick together. Take a small amount into each hand (a tablespoonful approximately) and, starting with one foot, work the salt onto the skin as you come up the leg, using up-and-down and circular motions.

Try to rub firmly, even vigorously, on skin that is usually exposed (such as the arms). Make sure that all of your skin is treated to some salt and rubbing. Work up each leg and then do each arm. Next, work salt into the skin around your back without straining yourself (this is where a partner comes in handy). Then apply the salt (rubbing firmly but not irritatingly) to the abdomen and chest and up to the neck (avoid breast tissues).

After the salt rub you need to shower, ideally using a hand shower and warm water to cleanse the surface of the skin As you are doing this and the water is playing on a given area, use your free hand to rub the salt and water off the skin, giving the area a bit more friction as you do so. Dry with a vigorous towelling down and go to bed (make sure it and the room is warm). You should sleep very well. The first few times you use the Salt Glow you may perspire heavily. Have water by the bed in case you get thirsty. As your skin becomes more efficient, this heavy perspiration will lessen.

Epsom Salts Bath

There are few more effective ways of stimulating skin function than an Epsom salts bath. It dramatically increases elimination through the skin and is ideal if there is any tendency towards acidity or rheumatic problems, or if there is a need to detoxify (this applies to almost everyone nowadays, see chapter 7). This method should *not* be used by anyone with a serious cardiac condition or diabetes, or with an 'open' or weeping skin condition.

The materials required for this treatment are one pound (340 grams) of commercial Epsom salts, a quarter to a half pound (85–170 grams) of sea salt and a dessertspoonful of iodine (choose the clear variety to avoid staining the bath). All ingredients should be widely available from good pharmacies.

Place the ingredients into a comfortably hot bath. This combination of salts and iodine approximates the constituents of the sea. Stay in the bath for not less than ten minutes and not more than twenty. All you have to do is lie there as it is quite impossible to wash in this salt mixture. If you stay in beyond ten minutes, top the bath up with hot water. When you get out do not shower – just towel yourself dry and get into a pre-warmed bed. As with the Salt Glow, you should expect to sweat heavily – and to sleep even more heavily. Have water by the bed as you may need to top up the lost liquid. In the morning take a shower and apply a moisturizer to the skin as a whole.

It is not recommended that you take an Epsom salts bath more than once a week. Once a month is probably the ideal for general detoxification purposes and stimulation of skin function.

The Peat Bath

When you use peat in a bath you are adding the combined concentrated material of hundreds of thousands of years of compression of the organic materials from decaying mosses, leaves and roots. The resulting 'soup' contains rich supplies of silica, sulphur, iron, resins and many minerals and harmless acids. Many of these ingredients help to neutralize harmful toxins on and under the skin, and since many of the micro-elements in peat can be absorbed through the skin, these can also influence your general health. A peat bath can be particularly beneficial to skin problems (although medical research has also shown that it can help rheumatic and blood pressure problems, circulatory difficulties and in restoring balance when there are sugar disturbances).

The best way of using peat is to apply it as a paste to the body surface as a whole. While this can be done effectively at health spas, it is not a practical proposition in the home. By using liquid (Austrian) peat (obtainable at any pharmacy and most health stores) you can enjoy the health benefits of peat in your own bathroom.

All you need do is pour the liquid (amounts will be indicated on the container) into a hot bath and soak for 20–30 minutes. You need to shower well afterwards and retire to a warm bed. As in the case of the Salt Glow and Epsom salts bath, you might expect to perspire more than usual that night and sleep very well indeed. Have water by your bed to make up the liquid lost through sweating, and be prepared to change your sheets next morning.

How often should you take a peat bath? This depends on your needs. If you just want to experience peat and give your skin a boost from its wonderful ingredients, then once or twice a month is adequate.

Sauna

Unless you are lucky enough to have a sauna at home this needs to be a treat you give yourself when you go along to a local health club or sauna bath. In the wood-lined room of the traditional Scandinavian sauna you are exposed to a dry-heat bath which induces a great deal of perspiration.

The effects are profound. Most people experience a great deal of stress release and relaxation along with the enormous elimination produced via the sweating. The benefits to circulation are well researched and proven, and anyone with a skin problem can be sure there will be an improvement after the skin has opened in the dry heat. Muscular and joint aches and stiffness are relieved and breathing problems also benefit.

Circulation is even further enhanced if the skin is stimulated during the sauna. You do not have to use birch twigs in the way the Finnish people do – you can just briskly rub the skin with a loofah or bath-mitt every now and then while sitting in the sauna. If you are not used to sauna you should stick to a 20-minute introduction followed by a tepid shower (or a cold one – the Finns dive into snow after theirs!) and a full-body massage.

One sauna a month is a wonderful aid to regular detoxification and skin cleansing – more often if you like but probably not more than once a week. When taking a sauna, follow this routine:

1 A short, warm shower followed by 10–15 minutes in the sauna.
2 A 30-second cool or cold plunge (many saunas have plunge baths available for this purpose) or shower. A few minutes' rest in a warm room is a good idea at this time.
3 Another 10–15 minutes in the sauna is indicated once you are used to the process, and this should again be followed by a cool shower or plunge, and a rest.
4 A massage after this rounds off a super indulgence which will do wonders for you and your skin.

When you are in the sauna you will notice benches. The ones nearest the ceiling are the hottest ones. By adapting to the lower bench first and only moving to the higher ones later, you let your body acclimatize to what is a novel experience for most of us. Do not eat for an hour before or after a sauna if you can help it, but replenish with liquid whenever you feel the need. Take medical advice before using a sauna if you have any serious medical condition, especially diabetes or a heart complaint.

A FINAL TIP

Inversion – lying in a position in which the head is lower than the body – has been shown to help restore circulation to the head/scalp and to increase hair growth. Take care not to do this if you have high blood pressure or eye problems such as glaucoma. Inversion or slant boards are available which allow you to strap your ankles to the elevated end with the head hanging well below the level of the feet. Fifteen minutes of this daily works wonders for scalp and hair quality.

CHAPTER NINE

Other Scalp Problems

Apart from dandruff there are a number of common problems that can affect the scalp. These include alopaecia, psoriasis, ringworm and head lice. This chapter looks at ways of treating these conditions, including self-help methods.

Some problems that can produce hair loss or scalp irritation are actually self-inflicted, or may be the result of actions by inexperienced or inefficient hairdressers. The way hair is cared for (or not cared for) and the many things done in the name of 'beauty' and fashion have much to answer for. It is suggested that you carefully read the advice on this topic in chapter 8.

As this chapter gives advice on aromatherapy oils and other applications, please bear in mind that it is important that you test these first in case you are sensitive to any of them. A skin-patch test is the easy answer. Apply a little of the substance to a patch of normal, healthy skin (on the forearm for example), and cover this with sticking plaster for some hours. When you remove the plaster, assess whether the skin has become irritated where the oil or substance was applied. If so, do not use it on the scalp or skin.

ALOPAECIA AND HAIR LOSS

Many factors contribute to balding (alopaecia), which is so common in males as to almost be the norm. When baldness is unnatural, with the hair suddenly falling out in tufts and patches, the condition is called alopaecia areata. This situation, which is also more common among men, is very distressing for the sufferer, especially as there seems little that medical science (conventional or alternative) can offer apart from sympathy and general advice.

Medical treatment for alopaecia often involves the use of drugs. Some of these do actually produce hair regrowth, although this tends to be fluffy and light and to fall out again as soon as the drug is stopped. Side-effects are common.

The causes of alopaecia are unknown, although there is often a degree of emotional distress in the background well before the hair starts to fall out. There may also be a link with hormonal imbalances, specific medical conditions or nutrient deficiencies. In some instances there are obvious reasons – the use of particular medications or treatments such as radiotherapy, for example. More commonly, however, such baldness patterns are not patchy (as in alopecia areata) but are simply 'male pattern baldness', or a gradual thinning of the hair in women past the menopause.

The good news about alopecia areata is that the hair usually grows back on its own, within a few months of falling out, whatever treatment is given – although it might grow back with a different colour. The bad news is that the bald patches may recur, or new ones develop, with little warning. Sometimes the hair-loss pattern involves eyebrows and eyelashes as well as the head (and even body) hair, which is even more distressing. This is called alopecia universalis.

Self-treatment

One of the first steps in treating hair loss is to reduce levels of stress. Advice should be sought from someone who can instruct you in breathing and relaxation techniques. If appropriate, psychotherapy should also be considered.

Stress reduction should be combined with attention to diet. There are reports of long-term high-dosage zinc supplementation helping recovery from alopecia (Polish research) but this approach should only be attempted under expert supervision. Other nutrients that have been connected with alopecia include iron and the B-vitamin biotin, and these may be supplemented if needed, under supervision.

The third step is employ techniques to enhance circulation to and detoxification of the skin and scalp. Various essential oils have been suggested as helpful – although no clinical trials have been done to support the claims. They will certainly do no harm and might help, but should be diluted in a carrier oil such as almond, soya or sesame oil before being applied to the skin. Try massaging either lavender oil or a blend of one part rosemary to two parts almond oil into the scalp daily. An alternative approach from Ayurvedic medicine is to massage warm bhringaraj oil or brahmi oil into the scalp daily. All of these oils should be available from pharmacies and health stores.

A naturopathic approach is to massage vitamin E oil into the scalp nightly. Then, for two weeks, follow this pattern: for two nights in a row massage castor oil into the scalp for ten minutes and then cover with a hot, damp towel for 30 minutes. Follow this by covering the head with a plastic shower cap and sleeping in it overnight. In the morning shampoo gently, and rinse with apple cider vinegar. For the next two nights do the same thing using olive oil instead of castor oil, and the following two nights use wheatgerm oil. Have a day's rest before repeating the process for six nights. Then go back to the vitamin E oil every night. Repeat the intensive cycle as above every few months if the problem persists

Dead Sea products can be used with some success if the hair follicles are still alive. The method used is similar to that described in the treatment of psoriasis (see below).

PSORIASIS

This unsightly and distressing (sometimes very itchy) scaly skin condition can manifest itself in different ways. Although it does not always involve the scalp, this is where it is most likely to be found. Psoriasis can look very much like dandruff or it may involve the entire scalp, with either fine or extremely thick flaky, red patches and scales. Psoriasis affects men and women equally, usually starting between the ages of 15 and 30.

Medical treatment usually involves topical applications of different materials. Most commonly, these are tar-based and oil-based creams and lotions, but creams containing hydrocortisone are also used. All such treatments should be under the direction of a dermatologist. Together with ultraviolet light, these treatments can help to provide short-term relief and to keep the condition under control. None of these approaches cures the condition, however, which remains a stubbornly resistant problem for many people throughout their lives.

Dead Sea Therapy

In Israel, a special method for treating psoriasis has

been developed. Using various products from the Dead Sea as well as the sunshine of that special area, the treatment has received excellent reports of success. The salt from the Dead Sea is not just any old sea salt – it consists of an extraordinary concentration of substances such as potassium and magnesium – and it is virtually free of all pollutants. These salts seem to draw toxins from below skin lesions and have a remarkable soothing and healing quality – claims which are amply supported by hundreds of research studies. The salts are available at most health-food shops.

You can use Dead Sea products to treat your own psoriasis. If the condition is mild or the flakes thin and not very adherent to the scalp, use Dead Sea Shampoo (for dry hair), applying the shampoo from the bottle neat onto the scalp, and creating a lather using a little water. Do this every day for a week at least, ensuring that the lather stays on the scalp for not less than 10 minutes before washing off. Slowly reduce the frequency of treatments until you use the special shampoo only twice weekly.

For more severe psoriasis of the scalp treat the head with Dead Sea mud, letting it stay in place for 15 minutes before washing off using Dead Sea shampoo. Do this daily for a week and then slowly reduce frequency until you apply mud and shampoo only twice weekly. You can also use this method to treat alopaecia.

Self-treatment using Dead Sea products in a 'neutral' bath can also be helpful. This means soaking for up to 45 minutes in a bath at body temperature in which a pound or more of sea salt (ideally Dead Sea salt) has been dissolved. Pat dry afterwards and go to bed. Do this daily during acute psoriasis episodes which affect the body skin. If the scalp is also affected, make sure that as much of it as possible is immersed.

You can start to use any of the methods described above as soon as you sense that a recurrence of psoriasis is about to happen. The condition may seem more 'angry' than usual for the first day or two of treatment, but this is a positive sign.

Nutritional Therapy

British nutritional experts, Drs Stephen Davis and Alan Stewart, set out a dietary strategy for treating psoriasis in their book *Nutritional Medicine*. They recommend a severe reduction in animal fats at the same time as an increase in fruit and vegetable intake.

Zinc is recommended as a supplement, with 30–40 mg daily being the suggested dose. The doctors stress, however, that this supplementation should be carried out under the direction of a medical adviser as there are some risks of unbalancing other nutrients if high zinc supplementation is prolonged – and the condition is unlikely to respond in a short time.

From the United States, Professor Melvyn Werbach reports on a number of nutritional strategies that have been found helpful in treating psoriasis in general.(See his book *Nutritional Influences on Illness*, Thorsons.) These include supplements of vitamins A and B_{12} (by injection into skin lesions), folic acid, zinc, selenium, essential fatty acids and lecithin. Careful supplementation under the guidance of a nutrition expert is called for to make sense of the various possible strategies that might be used.

There are also reports of food sensitivities relating to psoriasis. Where elimination diets have been introduced, one case revealed that fruits – especially citrus – nuts, corn and milk were causing the problem. Other cases pinpointed acidic foods such as tomato, coffee, pineapple and soda. Clearly these were individually devised programmes, and self-assessment and treatment could prove difficult. Wheat sensitivity is a common finding in psoriasis conditions, and a period of exclusion lasting not less than a month is needed to assess the impact of this avoidance pattern on the skin condition. Again it must be emphasized that expert help rather than do-it-yourself approaches are called for.

One strong clue as to which foods might be influencing the condition can be found by listing whatever was eaten about 24 hours before acute eruptions of the condition or increased itchiness, Careful detective work can help to identify culprit foods which should be eliminated for the time being.

Other studies show the benefits in treating

psoriasis with regime of fasting or eating only vegetarian foods. These trials may have been successful due to the allergy-causing foods that were being eliminated, or perhaps because of the detoxification and reduction of inflammation-enhancing substances found in non-vegetarian diets.

What becomes clear from the evidence available from nutritional research is that, while there is no single pattern which helps all patients, a number of tactics are worth trying.

Herbal Treatments

American experts suggest taking a teaspoonful of herbal tincture, containing equal parts of sarsaparilla, burdock and cleavers, three times a day. Sarsaparilla in particular seems to help by 'binding' bacterial toxins in the intestines, which is another piece of evidence supporting the value of a dietary and detoxification approach to the condition.

Aromatherapy

A variety of aromatherapy (essential) oils have been used to treat psoriasis including geranium, juniper, lavender and tea tree. These can be used in a bath simply by adding seven to eight drops neat into warm water. Alternatively, you can use them in a compress over a skin lesion. To do this, add five or six drops to a basin of hot water, and place some lint and lace on the surface of the water to absorb the essential oils and some water. Ring this out lightly and place over the lesion, bandaging it to keep it secure for 15–30 minutes before replacing it.

The essential oils can also be massaged into the area after they have been added to a suitable 'carrier' oil. Choose two or three of the oils listed on page 101 and blend two drops of each into a teaspoonful of almond or another carrier oil. Massage lightly into the skin.

RINGWORM

This is a highly contagious fungal infection characterized by a circular or half-moon pattern of reddish colour with a pale centre. The edges of the arc or ring may be scaly and there may be blisters. The lesion will be very itchy indeed. When this appears on the scalp it is known as tinea capitis, and the result is a circular bald patch as the hair breaks off close to the scalp.

Children acquire the infection from pets (kittens and puppies especially) or from other children. Schools and playgroups commonly have someone with the condition most of the time – especially in the winter months – and episodes occur when almost all the children in a class or group are affected. When an outbreak occurs, a doctor should be consulted who may prescribe systemic medication along with topical creams. You should also use common-sense self-help measures, such as those mentioned below. Adults can also acquire the infection through contact with an infected person or animal. Many people with chronic yeast infections have ringworm outbreaks.

Systemic treatment of underlying yeast infections is often the only way of preventing constant recurrence of this problem, and the advice given regarding candidiasis (see Chapter 3) should be followed if ringworm occurs more than once. This can be combined with the conventional medical treatment prescribed by a doctor.

Dietary strategies for any fungal or yeast problem – systemic or local – should include a low sugar intake and supplementation with *L. acidophilus* and *Bifidobacteria* to help normalize the intestinal tract which may harbour yeast overgrowth. A local 'alternative' approach which is just as (or even more) successful than topical medication from the doctor involves bandaging a thin slice of garlic over the patch of fungal activity for several days.

Use of the essential oil of the tea tree is very useful for topical application of this or any fungal infection. It should be used daily several times (if the garlic approach is not used) until no sign of the redness, and no itching, remains.

HEAD LICE

Lice are parasites that live on the skin of the hairy parts of the body. Head lice, in particular, can cause inflammation and a great deal of irritation and itching as a result of their feeding pattern, which involves sucking blood through the skin.

The main way of acquiring lice is through contact with an infected individual – using his or her brushes or combs, sleeping or resting the head on cushions or furniture material where the infected head has rested, or by direct physical contact. Pubic lice can be caught by sexual contact or by using towels or bedding which has been in contact with an infected individual.

Anti-lice shampoos are available from all pharmacies. The shampoo should be applied and left in place for some minutes, after which the hair should be carefully combed with a metal comb to remove nits (louse eggs). The process may need to be repeated several times over a period of days until all signs of lice have gone. If anyone in the family is infected it is probably wise for everyone to have this treatment.

Apart from direct medication, strict hygiene is an important factor in preventing contagion or spread of lice. Using your own towels, brushes etc. to avoid cross-infection is essential.

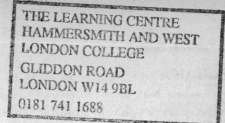

Index